PREGNANT WITH PCOS

The Effect of Polycystic Ovary Syndrome on Fertility and How to Manage Conception.

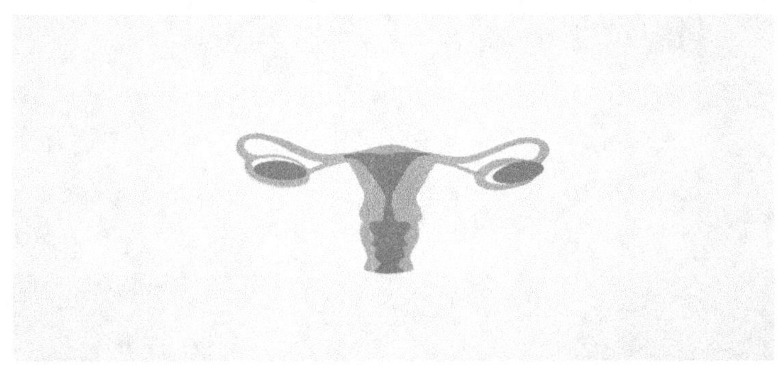

Terri Hogan

Copyright © 2024 by [Terri Hogan]

TABLE OF CONTENT

INTRODUCTION

PCOS is a prominent factor that affects the fertility journey of many people, making it a vital thread in the complex tapestry of reproductive health. The goal of this book, "Pregnant with PCOS," is to provide light on the special difficulties and victories encountered by people negotiating the complex relationship between PCOS and pregnancy.

PCOS, a hormonal condition that affects people who have ovaries, comes with a variety of challenges, such as irregular menstrual periods and insulin resistance. When people with PCOS decide to become parents, they frequently face difficult issues and doubts. This thorough guide aims to simplify the complicated issues surrounding PCOS by providing information on its causes, signs, and subtleties of diagnosis.

The book delves into the core of PCOS-related fertility issues and covers a wide range of subjects, from medical procedures that can facilitate conception to lifestyle changes that are essential for treating the illness. The path to pregnancy is not just physical; mental and emotional health are important factors as well, and this book explores the complex interactions between the physiological and emotional dimensions of the process.

"Pregnant with PCOS" is a source of empowerment as well as a resource. This book tries to provide people with PCOS with the knowledge and resiliency necessary to negotiate the maze of fertility, finally assisting them in realizing their aspirations of becoming parents, through educational chapters, personal tales, and professional guidance.

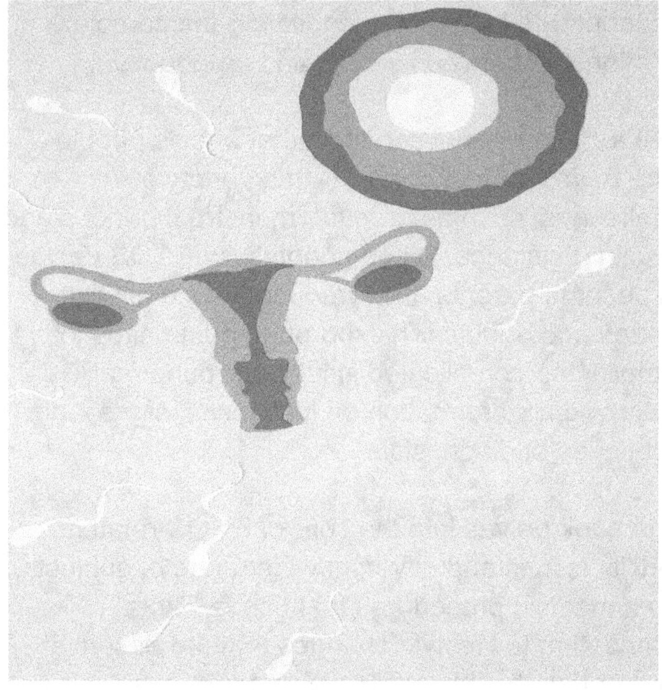

CHAPTER ONE

Understanding PCOS

What is PCOS?

Those with ovaries are susceptible to a common hormonal condition called polycystic ovarian syndrome, or PCOS. Its symptoms, which include irregular menstrual periods, ovarian cysts, and increased levels of androgens (male hormones), are caused by an imbalance in reproductive hormones. In addition to having an effect on insulin sensitivity and fertility, PCOS can cause physical symptoms like hirsutism (excessive hair growth) and acne. Although the precise origin of PCOS is unknown, genetics and insulin resistance are thought to be important factors. Medication, lifestyle modifications, and occasionally fertility therapies are all part of management.

Reasons and Danger Elements

Molecular Predisposition:

Given that PCOS often runs in families, there may be a hereditary component. People who have a family history of PCOS are more likely to get the illness.

Insulin Resistance:

Blood sugar-regulating hormone insulin may work less well in people with PCOS. This may result in increased insulin levels, which in turn may cause the ovaries to overproduce androgens, or male hormones.

An imbalance of hormones:

Reproductive hormone imbalance, especially an overabundance of androgens like testosterone, is a factor in PCOS. This interferes with the ovaries' regular operation, which impacts the release of eggs during the menstrual cycle.

Low-Grade Inflammation:

PCOS is connected with chronic inflammation, which may contribute to insulin resistance. Inflammation can interfere with ovarian function and aggravate symptoms.

Factors of Lifestyle:

Obesity, which is frequently associated with PCOS, can be exacerbated by sedentary lifestyle and poor nutritional habits. Obesity can exacerbate insulin resistance and hormonal abnormalities.

Ethnicity:

According to several research, some ethnic groups, such as South Asian and African American women, may be more prone to PCOS. More research, however, is required to determine the specific association.

Endocrine Disruptor Exposure:

Environmental factors, such as endocrine-disrupting chemical exposure, may contribute to the development of PCOS. These substances can disrupt hormonal equilibrium.

Understanding the origins and risk factors for PCOS lays the groundwork for managing and treating the condition, with lifestyle changes and focused medications aimed at minimizing the specific problems given by this complex hormonal imbalance.

PCOS Symptoms and Diagnosis

PCOS symptoms include:

Menstrual Cycle Disruptions:

One of the distinguishing features is irregular periods. Women with PCOS may have sporadic or delayed menstrual periods, or sometimes no menstruation at all.

Ovarian Dysfunction:

PCOS can cause ovulation problems, resulting in infertility. Ovulatory dysfunction can cause infertility or trouble conceiving.

Hyperandrogenism:

Elevated androgen levels, such as testosterone, can cause acne, hirsutism (excessive hair growth, particularly on the face), and male-pattern baldness.

Polycystic Ovary Syndrome:

Individuals with PCOS may have several tiny cysts visible on ultrasonography of their ovaries. However, not all women with PCOS have polycystic ovaries, and the presence of cysts is not enough to diagnose the condition.

Insulin Deficiency:

Insulin resistance is widespread in PCOS, and it contributes to metabolic problems. This can result in weight gain, particularly around the abdomen.

Mood Swings:

Some people with PCOS may experience mood swings, anxiety, or sadness as a result of hormonal imbalances.

PCOS Diagnosis:

Physical Exam and Medical History:

A healthcare professional will ask about menstruation history and symptoms, as well as perform a physical exam to look for indicators of androgen excess, such as hirsutism or acne.

Tests on the blood:

Hormone levels in the blood are measured via blood tests, which include androgens, oestrogen, and insulin. PCOS is characterized by elevated androgen levels, particularly testosterone.

Ultrasound of the Pelvis:

To see the ovaries, a transvaginal ultrasound may be performed. Polycystic ovaries might have numerous tiny follicles and appear larger.

Other Conditions Excluded:

Because certain PCOS symptoms coincide with those of other illnesses, healthcare providers may order testing to rule out other causes of the symptoms.

PCOS diagnosis necessitates a multifaceted strategy that includes clinical, hormonal, and imaging evaluations. Early detection and care of PCOS are critical for alleviating symptoms, avoiding complications, and promoting reproductive health.

CHAPTER TWO

Navigating Fertility Challenges

PCOS and Fertility

For people with Polycystic Ovary Syndrome (PCOS), embarking on the path to parenting can be a perplexing process. This common hormonal disease, characterized by reproductive hormone abnormalities, can have a substantial impact on fertility and present particular complications.

Irregular ovulation is at the heart of PCOS-related reproductive issues. Because of hormonal abnormalities, the ovaries may not release eggs on a regular basis, making conception difficult. Fertility tracking becomes a delicate ballet with unpredictable menstrual cycles, demanding an intimate knowledge of ovulation patterns. This irregularity can be a cause of frustration and uncertainty for people attempting to conceive.

Insulin resistance, a prevalent side effect of PCOS, complicates the reproductive landscape even further. Elevated insulin levels might make it difficult to maintain a healthy weight and can interfere with ovulation. Lifestyle changes, such as eating a balanced diet and exercising regularly, are frequently included into fertility control.

On this path, medical interventions provide hope. Fertility therapies can be designed to address the specific issues posed by PCOS, ranging from ovulation-inducing drugs to assisted reproductive technologies such as in vitro fertilisation (IVF). These therapies are intended to improve ovulation and increase the likelihood of successful conception.

The emotional toll of PCOS-related fertility issues, however, should not be overlooked. The trek is not just physical, but also deeply personal and frequently emotionally charged. Professional and personal support networks are critical in navigating the emotional ups and downs of fertility treatments.

Each chapter of the story of PCOS and fertility is a tribute to tenacity and optimism. Despite the difficulties, many people with PCOS are able to conceive and enjoy the benefits of motherhood. This narrative strives to empower folks on this journey by unravelling the complexities of PCOS and fertility, offering insights, compassion, and a route to realising the ambition of starting a family.

PCOS Treatment Options

Changes in Lifestyle:

Changes in Diet: A balanced, low-glycemic diet can help manage insulin resistance, a typical feature of PCOS.

Regular Exercise: Physical activity helps with weight management, insulin sensitivity, and overall well-being.
Medications:

Birth Control Pills: They regulate menstrual cycles and lower testosterone levels.
Anti-androgen medications are used to treat symptoms such as acne and hirsutism.
Metformin improves insulin sensitivity, especially in people who have insulin resistance.

Treatments for Infertility:

Ovulation-Inducing Medications: To stimulate ovulation, clomiphene citrate or letrozole may be administered.

IVF (In Vitro Fertilisation): Assisted reproductive technique in which an egg is fertilised with sperm outside of the body.

Surgery:

Ovarian Drilling: A surgical treatment that involves making microscopic holes in the ovaries in order to encourage regular ovulation.

Weight Control:

Achieving and maintaining a healthy weight can help to alleviate symptoms and improve the efficacy of other treatments.

Alternative Therapies:

Acupuncture: Acupuncture has helped some people find relief from PCOS symptoms and enhanced fertility.

While evidence is limited, certain herbs may be used to alleviate symptoms, but it is critical to speak with a healthcare physician first.

Specific Symptom Management:

Dermatological treatments for acne or excessive hair growth that address the cosmetic features of PCOS.

Hair Removal procedures: To treat hirsutism, many procedures such as laser hair removal or electrolysis may be utilised.

Monitoring and follow-up on a regular basis:

Continuous monitoring of symptoms and hormone levels allows treatment strategies to be adjusted as needed.

PCOS treatment is frequently tailored to the individual, taking into account symptoms, goals (such as controlling PCOS for fertility or symptom relief), and overall health. Individuals with PCOS receive comprehensive and personalized therapy through a collaborative approach comprising healthcare practitioners from multiple specialties, including endocrinologists, gynecologists, and fertility specialists.

Managing Emotional and Mental Health with PCOS:

PCOS has an influence that extends beyond the physical sphere, weaving into the intricate fabric of emotional and mental well-being. For people suffering from PCOS, the journey is more than just a physical one; it is a kaleidoscope of emotions, resilience, and self-discovery.

Influence on Self-Esteem:

Acne, hirsutism, and weight swings are physical manifestations of PCOS that might challenge social beauty standards, potentially leading to a drop in self-esteem. The path to self-acceptance becomes an important aspect of the emotional landscape.

Obstacles to Fertility:

Fertility uncertainty and obstacles can elicit a wide range of emotions, from optimism and anticipation to disappointment and despair. Fertility treatments may bring an additional degree of emotional complication to the experience.

Body Image Issues:

The impact of PCOS on weight and body composition can contribute to body image issues. Balancing the desire for a healthy lifestyle with society pressures necessitates a fine balance.

Anxiety and Stress:

Stress and anxiety can be exacerbated by the chronic nature of PCOS and its possible impact on daily living. It is critical for overall well-being to manage these emotional responses.

Relationship Effects:

The emotional toll of infertility issues or mood changes connected with PCOS symptoms may have an impact on intimate relationships. Communication is crucial, as is mutual support.

Knowledge Gives You Power:

Understanding PCOS and its various symptoms allows people to take control of their health. Education becomes a pillar for traversing the emotional environment, cultivating a sense of control and resilience.

Networks of Support:

Creating a strong support network, whether through friends, family, or online forums, gives a secure area for people to discuss their experiences and seek understanding. Connecting with those who have gone through similar experiences can be emotionally beneficial.

Assistance from a Professional:

Professionals in mental health play an important role in giving tools and coping methods. Stress, anxiety, and the emotional complexity associated with PCOS can all benefit from therapeutic interventions.

Emotional and mental well-being is an important chapter in the story of PCOS. It entails acknowledging one's emotional environment, practicing self-compassion, and cultivating resilience. Individuals with PCOS construct an emotional tapestry as they traverse the peaks and valleys of their journey, demonstrating strength, courage, and the transformational power of self-care.

CHAPTER THREE

Lifestyle Modifications

Nutrition and PCOS

Nutrition is essential to PCOS treatment since metabolic variables and PCOS are closely related. Making healthy food choices can increase insulin sensitivity, lessen symptoms, and make PCOS sufferers feel better overall.

A balanced intake of macronutrients

Strive for a diet that is well-balanced in terms of carbohydrates, proteins, and fats. Lean proteins, complex carbs, and healthy fats are good sources of nutrients that can help control insulin resistance and keep blood sugar levels steady.

Glycemic Index Meal Plan:

If you want to avoid unanticipated blood sugar spikes, give low-glycemic foods first consideration. Legumes, whole grains, and non-starchy veggies make up this.

Regular Meals and Snacks:

Smaller, more balanced meals can help control blood sugar and insulin levels throughout the day. Cutting down on long stretches of time without food is essential to managing the metabolic aspects of PCOS.

Reducing Sugar Added and Processed Foods:

Reduce your intake of processed meals, sugar-filled drinks, and refined carbohydrates. These might make PCOS symptoms worse and raise insulin resistance.

Healthful Fats:

Include healthy fat-containing foods such as avocados, nuts, seeds, and olive oil. In addition to producing hormones, these fats aid in the sensation of fullness.

High-Fibre Foods:

To enhance your fibre intake, eat more fruits, vegetables, and whole grains. Fibre helps control blood sugar levels, improve digestive health, and assist with weight management.

Consuming Protein in Moderation:

Include lean protein sources such tofu, fish, poultry, and lentils. Protein helps maintain muscle mass and improves a well-balanced diet.

Consuming an abundance of water

To stay adequately hydrated, sip on lots of water or herbal teas. Reducing cravings and enhancing general health are two benefits of drinking adequate water.

Conclusion:

If you believe taking specialised supplements like inositol, omega-3 fatty acids, or vitamin D would help you, consult a physician. These can further assist those who have PCOS.

Personalized Approach:

Individuals with PCOS may need to follow particular diets. Based on individual symptoms, lifestyle decisions, and health objectives, a qualified dietitian or nutritionist can provide customised guidance.

A comprehensive approach to diet, along with the required lifestyle adjustments and medication schedules, can help treat PCOS to the best of its abilities. It is advantageous for one's physical and emotional wellbeing to continuously make health-conscious judgements. In tackling the metabolic complexity connected to this intricate hormonal condition, it is also essential.

Exercise and Fitness for PCOS Patients

In order to manage polycystic ovarian syndrome (PCOS), regular exercise is crucial. Exercise has been demonstrated in numerous studies to assist individuals with PCOS feel better overall, control their symptoms, and enhance their metabolic health.

Increasing Insulin Sensitivity:

Regular exercise enhances insulin sensitivity, assisting in the control of blood sugar. For people with PCOS who may also be insulin resistant, this is really crucial.

Supporting the Control of Weight:

Physical activity plays a major role in weight management. Maintaining a healthy weight might reduce some PCOS symptoms and enhance hormonal balance.

Cardiovascular Exercise:

Getting your heart and muscles strong, your endurance up, and your weight down can all be achieved by walking, running, cycling, or swimming vigorously.

Strengthening Activities:

Resistance training, such as weightlifting and bodyweight workouts, can build muscle mass. Increased muscle mass is associated with improved weight management and a faster metabolism.

Interval-based training:

HIIT, or high-intensity interval exercise, may be beneficial for PCOS patients. Interspersing short bursts of intensive activity with rest periods can increase both insulin sensitivity and cardiovascular fitness.

Lowering Tension:

Working out is one of the best methods to reduce stress. Including yoga or meditation in your exercise regimen can help maintain hormonal and emotional balance, which can help reduce stress and its associated symptoms, such as PCOS.

Consistency Is The Key:

Exercise regularity and consistency are more important than intensity. Try to get in at least 150 minutes of moderate-intensity aerobic activity or 75 minutes of vigorous-intensity aerobic activity every week, along with two or more days of muscle-strengthening exercises.

Personalized Approach:

Adapt the workout regimen to the individual's needs and physical state. Consult a healthcare professional or fitness specialist to design a personalised strategy that takes your goals and health into consideration.

Social Services:

Peer assistance during group activities, such as workouts, helps keep the activity consistent and add to its enjoyment.

Keeping an eye on developments

Keep track of your exercise and development. This not only helps to adjust the training regimen as needed, but it also acts as motivation.

Patients with PCOS who regularly include exercise into their lifestyle can benefit from its transforming potential. Whether the objective is to manage weight, lower stress levels, or enhance metabolic health, the all-encompassing advantages of exercise play a substantial role in the entire approach to managing PCOS.

PCOS Stress Reduction

Stress management is a critical component of treating the multiple issues linked to polycystic ovarian syndrome (PCOS). Having good stress management skills is crucial for overall health since chronic stress can worsen symptoms and disrupt hormone balance.

Practices of Mindfulness and Meditation:

Two methods that can ease stress and encourage calmness are mindfulness meditation and deep breathing exercises. By applying these techniques to everyday tasks, emotional stability is enhanced.

Frequent Exercise:

Getting your hands dirty is a great way to relax. Regular exercise releases endorphins, the body's natural mood boosters, whether it be from weight training, yoga, or cardiovascular sports.

Adequate Rest:

To improve your general well-being and stress tolerance, make obtaining enough sleep a top priority. Establishing a calm nighttime routine and adhering to it will help you practise better sleep hygiene.

Social Services:

Developing relationships with family, friends, or support networks is a beneficial means of sharing experiences and getting emotional support. Strong social bonds can mitigate the damaging consequences of stress.

Efficient Time Management:

Sort up your chores and set priorities for your tasks. Dividing challenging jobs into smaller, more doable chunks could make them less intimidating and unpleasant.

An alimentative diet

Maintain a balanced diet, placing special emphasis on nutrient-dense foods. Consuming a nutritious diet enhances stress tolerance and improves both physical and mental health.

Cognitive-Behavioral Methods:

Cognitive-behavioral therapy (CBT) assists people in recognising and altering harmful thought patterns and behaviours, which can help them manage stress.

Creative Recess:

Take part in artistic, musical, or literary endeavours. These channels offer a way for one to express oneself and can be used as therapeutic stress-reduction methods.

Limiting the Input:

Limit your consumption of stimulants like alcohol and caffeine because they can raise your stress and anxiety levels.

Getting Expert Assistance:

If stress is too much for you to handle, think about getting help from a mental health specialist. Counsellors or therapists can offer coping mechanisms that are customised to meet each person's needs.

Understanding how stress and PCOS are related is essential to holistic management. Effective stress management practices can help people with PCOS become more resilient, improve their general mental health, and provide the groundwork for overcoming the difficulties brought on by this complicated hormonal condition.

CHAPTER FOUR

Medical Interventions

Medications for PCOS

Multiple drugs are frequently used in the medical care of Polycystic Ovary Syndrome (PCOS) in order to target specific symptoms and underlying hormonal abnormalities. The selection of medication is contingent upon the specific symptoms, intended fertility, and general health. To ascertain the best course of action, it is imperative to speak with a healthcare professional. The following list of common drugs is used to treat PCOS:

Contraceptives by mouth:

Oestrogen and progesterone-containing birth control tablets lower testosterone levels, control menstrual cycles, and treat acne and hirsutism symptoms.

Anti-Androgen Supplements:

In order to lessen the impact of androgens and assist control symptoms like acne and excessive hair growth, doctors may prescribe flutamide or spirolactone.

Drugs that Sensitise to Insulin:

It's common practice to prescribe metformin to increase insulin sensitivity. In certain situations, it can increase fertility, decrease testosterone levels, and control menstrual cycles.

Drugs that Induce Ovulation:

The medications letrozole and clomiphene citrate induce ovulation and are frequently used to help PCOS-affected women become pregnant.

Treatments for Fertility:

For those whose infertility is connected to PCOS, in vitro fertilisation (IVF) or other assisted reproductive technologies may be suggested as a means of conception assistance.

Medication for Weight Loss:

When lifestyle modifications alone are not enough to manage PCOS, prescription drugs for weight loss may be taken into consideration as part of a holistic strategy.

Hormone Treatment:

In some circumstances, gonadotropin-releasing hormone (GnRH) agonists or antagonists may be administered to control menstrual cycles and ovulation.

Supplements with Inositol:

One kind of B-vitamin that has been researched is isothiol; it may help improve ovarian function and insulin sensitivity in PCOS patients. It comes in several forms, including D-chiro-inositol and myo-inositol.

Supplements of vitamin D:

It's possible for some PCOS sufferers to be vitamin D deficient. It could be advised to use vitamin D supplements to treat this deficit and promote general health.

Medication for Pain:

In certain instances, nonsteroidal anti-inflammatory medications (NSAIDs) may be used to treat discomfort related to illnesses such ovarian cysts.

It's important to remember that not everyone with PCOS will need pharmaceutical interventions, and that the choice of drugs depends on specific conditions. Effective PCOS management involves routine monitoring, honest communication with healthcare professionals, and a comprehensive strategy that combines medication with lifestyle changes.

PCOS and Assisted Reproductive Technologies (ART)

When it comes to overcoming infertility issues, Assisted Reproductive Technologies (ART) are essential for those with Polycystic Ovary Syndrome (PCOS). ART refers to a range of cutting-edge medical procedures intended to support conception in situations where natural approaches are difficult or unsuccessful. The following are important ART choices for PCOS patients:

IVF, or in vitro fertilisation:

An egg is fertilised externally with sperm during in vitro fertilisation (IVF). IVF can improve the odds of successful conception for PCOS patients who may experience ovulatory disruption.

Induction of Ovulation:

It is possible to administer drugs like letrozole or clomiphene citrate to induce ovulation. For those with PCOS who are attempting to get pregnant, this is frequently the first course of action.

IUI, or intrauterine insemination:

During the woman's reproductive window, sperm are directly inserted into the uterus during an IUI procedure. It is occasionally used with drugs that stimulate ovulation.

Sensation of the Ovaries:

IVF or IUI cycles may include ovarian stimulation. Fertility drugs increase the likelihood of a successful fertilisation by stimulating the ovaries to generate numerous eggs.

Drilling of Polycystic Ovary:

Small incisions are made in the ovaries during this surgical technique to trigger ovulation. It is taken into consideration for PCOS patients who don't react well to other forms of reproductive treatment.

Genetic testing prior to implantation (PGT):

To improve the chances of a healthy pregnancy, PGT can be used in conjunction with IVF to test embryos for genetic abnormalities prior to implantation.

Freezing of Egg or Embryo:

When undergoing reproductive treatments, PCOS patients may decide to store their eggs or embryos for later use. This is especially important for people who are worried about how age affects fertility.

Changes in Lifestyle:

Lifestyle changes such as nutrition, exercise, and stress reduction can enhance fertility treatments and enhance overall reproductive health, even though they are not a conventional ART.

It's critical to approach ART from a complete and individualised standpoint, taking into account each person's unique needs and circumstances. The choice to pursue ART is frequently made in consultation with one's medical team as well as the person or couple. Success rates can differ. When combining ART with PCOS management, routine monitoring, honest communication, and emotional support are essential parts of the process.

Options for PCOS Surgery

While surgical interventions are rarely the primary choice for treating Polycystic Ovary Syndrome (PCOS), they could be taken into consideration in some situations when non-surgical treatments have failed. The following are a few PCOS surgical options:

Laparoscopic ovarian diathermy, or ovarian drilling:

A minimally invasive laparoscopic method is used in ovarian drilling. By decreasing the synthesis of androgens, tiny holes are created on the ovarian surface, which may aid in the restoration of regular ovulation. When ovulation-inducing drugs such as letrozole or clomiphene citrate are ineffective, this method is taken into consideration.

Thyroid Wedge Excision:

In the past, improving ovulatory performance required removing a piece of the ovary during ovarian wedge resection. However, the availability of less invasive options has made this operation less commonplace in modern times.

Cystectomy:

Cystectomy may be necessary for PCOS patients who develop large ovarian cysts that hurt or result in other issues. In order to preserve the healthy ovarian tissue, cysts must be removed.

Tubal Ligation:

A permanent method of contraception called tubal ligation involves cutting or sealing the fallopian tubes. It's not a PCOS treatment, but it might be an option for those who are done having children and don't want to get pregnant.

It is important to remember that surgical treatments for PCOS are usually taken into consideration after all other forms of treatment have been tried or are deemed inappropriate for the patient. The decision to have any surgical operation should be carefully considered with a healthcare provider, taking into account the possible advantages and related complications. These surgeries are not without risk. Frequently, non-invasive methods like medication and lifestyle changes are given precedence over surgical procedures.

CHAPTER FIVE

Pregnancy with PCOS

Preconception Care for PCOS

Planning to conceive with Polycystic Ovary Syndrome (PCOS) requires preconception care. Prenatal health optimisation improves pregnancy outcomes and reduces problems. Important preconception care considerations for PCOS:

Regular checkups:

Schedule a preconception appointment with a doctor to examine health, discuss PCOS management, and address reproductive issues.

Weight Optimisation:

Weight control is essential for fertility and pregnancy safety. Management of weight can improve hormonal balance and ovulatory function.

Balanced Diet:

Balanced, nutrient-rich diet. Focus on complete foods, lean proteins, fruits, veggies, and whole grains. Consider consulting a qualified dietitian for personalized nutritional guidance.

Supplements:

Start taking prenatal vitamins with folic acid before conception. Adequate folic acid minimises the likelihood of neural tube abnormalities in the developing baby.

Blood Sugar Control:

If insulin resistance is a concern, consult with healthcare experts to regulate blood sugar levels with lifestyle adjustments or drugs like metformin.

Regular Exercise:

Engage in regular physical activity, which supports general health, helps manage weight, and adds to enhanced insulin sensitivity.

Manage Stress:

Incorporate stress management practices such as mindfulness, meditation, or yoga. Chronic stress can damage fertility and general well-being.

Quit smoking and restrict alcohol intake. Both smoking and heavy alcohol intake can significantly influence fertility and raise the chance of problems during pregnancy.

Regular Monitoring of Menstrual Cycles:

Track menstrual cycles to discover ovulation tendencies. This information can assist in optimizing the timing of conception attempts.

Consultation with Specialists:

If fertility issues persist, consider visiting with a fertility expert or reproductive endocrinologist to discuss assisted reproductive technology or other fertility therapies.

Preconception care is a collaborative effort involving the individual, their healthcare providers, and, if necessary, fertility specialists. It provides a foundation for a healthy pregnancy and boosts the odds of successful conception for those with PCOS.

Pregnancy Complications Associated with PCOS

While many individuals with Polycystic Ovary Syndrome (PCOS) go on to have healthy pregnancies, PCOS can raise the risk of certain problems. Regular prenatal care and regular monitoring by healthcare experts are critical for managing and reducing potential dangers. Here are several pregnancy complications connected with PCOS:

Gestational Diabetes:

Women with PCOS have an increased chance of acquiring gestational diabetes, a type of diabetes that arises during pregnancy. Regular blood glucose monitoring and lifestyle adjustments can help control this illness.

Preeclampsia:

PCOS may be connected with an enhanced chance of developing preeclampsia, a condition characterized by high blood pressure and severe organ damage. Close monitoring of blood pressure and other symptoms is crucial.

Preterm Birth:

There is a slightly greater risk of premature birth in pregnancies with women with PCOS. Early detection and management of risk factors contribute to minimising this risk.

Cesarean Section (C-Section):

The chance of necessitating a C-section may be raised in women with PCOS. This could be related to causes such as gestational diabetes, macrosomia (big baby), or other issues.

Gestational Hypertension:

Some persons with PCOS may face an increased risk of developing gestational hypertension, a disorder characterized by elevated blood pressure during pregnancy.

Miscarriage:

While the evidence is not conclusive, several studies imply a slightly greater risk of miscarriage in women with PCOS. Early prenatal treatment and monitoring can help identify and manage potential concerns.

Macrosomia (Large Baby):

Babies born to women with gestational diabetes associated with PCOS may be bigger than typical. This can raise the chance of difficulties during delivery.
Neonatal Intensive Care Unit (NICU)

Admission:

In some situations, infants born to moms with PCOS may require admission to the NICU, maybe due to difficulties related to prematurity or other causes.

It's important to highlight that these risks do not ensure difficulties, and many persons with PCOS have good pregnancies. Proactive prenatal care, including early and regular check-ups, monitoring of blood glucose levels, and communication with healthcare providers about any potential hazards, helps control and limit the effect of these issues. Each pregnancy is unique, and specific circumstances should determine the approach to care.

Postpartum Considerations for Individuals with PCOS

The postpartum period brings a series of specific considerations for those with Polycystic Ovary Syndrome (PCOS). Managing physical and emotional wellness during this time is critical. Here are some postpartum considerations:

Hormonal Changes:

Postpartum hormonal shifts may influence individuals with PCOS differently. Regular follow-ups with healthcare experts can help monitor hormone balance.

Lactation and Breastfeeding:

Some individuals with PCOS may have issues relating to lactation. Consultation with lactation professionals or healthcare practitioners can provide support and direction.

Blood Sugar Monitoring:

Individuals with a history of gestational diabetes or insulin resistance associated with PCOS should continue monitoring blood sugar levels afterward. Lifestyle adjustments may still be relevant.

Resumption of Menstrual Cycles:

Menstrual periods may take longer to return to normal. Women with PCOS may encounter irregularities, and resuming regular ovulation could differ.

Weight Management:

Postpartum weight management is critical for patients with PCOS. A balanced diet and gradual return to regular physical activity, under the advice of healthcare specialists, contribute to general well-being.

Contraception Choices:

Discuss contraception choices with healthcare experts, as individuals with PCOS may have special considerations. Some may adopt treatments that regulate menstrual cycles or assist manage symptoms.

Mental Health:

Postpartum mental wellness is vital. Individuals with PCOS may be at a higher risk for postpartum depression. Open contact with healthcare practitioners and seeking help from mental health specialists can be beneficial.

Reproductive Planning:

If considering subsequent pregnancies, it's crucial to discuss reproductive planning with healthcare experts. Preconception care, especially for women with PCOS, remains crucial for successive pregnancies.

Lifestyle Adjustments:

Balancing the pressures of new parenting with self-care is vital. Adequate sleep, a supportive environment, and stress management contribute to postpartum well-being.

Follow-Up with Specialists:

Continue follow-up meetings with experts, such as endocrinologists or reproductive endocrinologists, to address any persisting concerns connected to PCOS.

Navigating the postpartum period with PCOS demands a comprehensive and tailored approach. Open communication with healthcare providers, a focus on physical and emotional well-being, and support from family and friends provide a foundation for a good and joyful postpartum experience.

CHAPTER SIX

Success Stories

Actual experiences in life

Sure! I can give some broad narratives that people with PCOS may come across based on common elements, even if I don't have access to real-time or unique personal experiences:

Issues with Diagnosis:

A common problem amongst many PCOS sufferers is the difficulty in getting diagnosed. Before getting a conclusive diagnosis, symptoms like irregular periods or acne may be disregarded at first, frustrating the patient.

Influence on the Rate of Fertility

A number of people with PCOS talk about the psychological toll that infertility takes. Resilience and vulnerable periods coexist on the route to conception, which may entail a mix of medication, lifestyle modifications, and fertility therapies.

Managing Weight:

One recurrent topic is managing one's weight.
People frequently discuss how difficult it is to
balance lifestyle changes with PCOS symptoms,
emphasising the value of a customised approach to
nutrition and exercise.

Psychological Health:

A crucial component is mental and emotional
health. A few individuals relate to having
experienced mood swings, anxiety, or sadness
associated with hormone changes. In order to
overcome these obstacles, coping mechanisms
and support systems are essential.

Remarkable Achievements:

There are many inspiring tales of people with
PCOS who have managed the condition. These
stories frequently combine medical interventions
with lifestyle modifications and a proactive attitude
towards general health.

Teaching and Lobbying:

Many people go on to promote PCOS education
and awareness. By offering support to those going
through similar struggles, sharing stories online or
in groups helps dispel stigmas.

Postpartum Travels:

People with PCOS have a wide range of postpartum experiences. While some talk about the need for continued care and assistance during this crucial time, others share encouraging tales of successfully controlling symptoms.

Shifts in Lifestyle:

There are many success stories about changing one's lifestyle. People frequently talk about how their PCOS symptoms and general well-being are improved by dietary, exercise, and stress management modifications.

Making Your Way Through Healthcare

Finding medical professionals that are knowledgeable about PCOS is something that many people stress. Effective management is facilitated by cooperative connections with skilled specialists.

Networks of Support:

One theme that keeps coming up is creating or joining offline or online support networks. Developing ties with people who have gone through similar things as you does promotes a feeling of empowering community.

It is noteworthy that the experiences of individuals with PCOS vary, and strategies that are effective for one person might not be suitable for another. These stories emphasise resilience, the value of individualised care, and the complexity of the PCOS journey.

Advice from the Achievers

Sure! The following advice and viewpoints are from people who have effectively treated polycystic ovarian syndrome, or PCOS:

Knowledge is Power:

Make the time to familiarise yourself with PCOS. Making educated decisions about your health is made possible by having a thorough understanding of the illness, its symptoms, and the available treatments.

Stand up for Yourself:

Speak out for your own well-being. Find experts that genuinely understand and support your PCOS

journey and seek second views if you feel ignored
or misunderstood by healthcare practitioners.

Approaching a Holistic Lifestyle:

Adopt a comprehensive strategy for PCOS
management. Incorporate stress reduction, a
balanced diet, frequent exercise, and enough
sleep. Modest, long-lasting adjustments frequently
have a big impact.

Customised Dietary Interventions:

Create a customised nutrition plan by consulting
with a licenced nutritionist. You may control your
weight and enhance your general well-being by
customising your diet to your unique requirements
and tastes.

Regular Workout Schedule:

Create and follow a regular workout schedule. This
helps with overall health and insulin sensitivity in
addition to helping with weight management.

The Mind-Body Link

Examine mind-body techniques like meditation and
yoga. Stress management is essential for PCOS
patients, and these techniques can promote a
healthy mind-body link.

Frequent surveillance and examinations:

Continue to take charge of your health. Monitoring PCOS symptoms and getting regular checkups might help spot changes or possible problems early on.

Establish a Network of Support:

Make contact with other PCOS sufferers. A place to share stories, trade advice, and get support can be found in online communities, local meet-ups, or support groups.

Honour Little Victories:

Celebrate your little accomplishments along the way as you navigate PCOS. Acknowledging progress is a source of motivation, whether it be for sustaining a good habit or reaching a specific objective.

Relationships with Open Communication:

Discuss PCOS and its possible effects on fertility with your partner in a relationship in an open and honest manner. Having your partner's support and understanding can be quite beneficial.

Knowledge of Fertility:

Learn about your menstrual cycles and ovulation patterns if achieving fertility is your goal. You can improve the timing of conception by keeping track of your cycles.

Expert Counselling:

Consult medical specialists in gynaecology, endocrinology, or reproductive health for advice. Working with trained specialists guarantees a thorough and informed approach to PCOS management.

Recall that managing PCOS is very individualised, so what works for one person might not be appropriate for another. Success is on identifying a customised strategy that complements your lifestyle and health objectives.

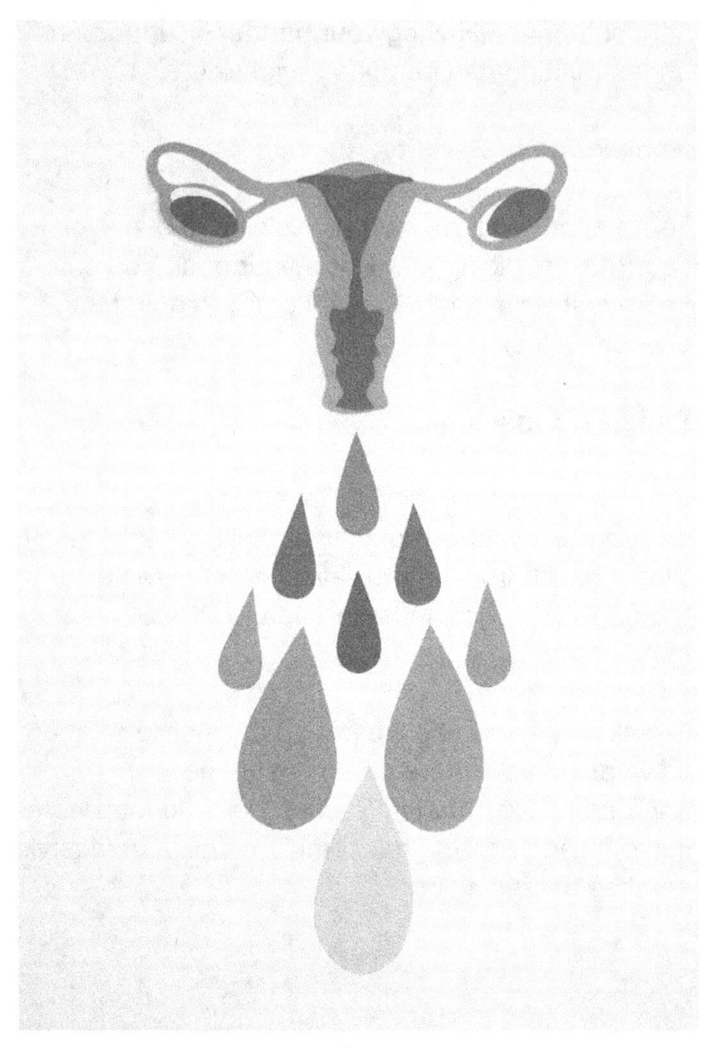

CHAPTER SEVEN

Resources and Support

Support Groups for PCOS

Finding support from others who share similar experiences can be valuable in navigating the challenges of Polycystic Ovary Syndrome (PCOS). Here are some avenues to explore for PCOS support groups:

Online Communities:

Platforms like Reddit, Facebook, and health forums often host PCOS-specific groups. Joining these online communities allows you to connect with individuals globally, sharing insights and support.

PCOS Organizations:

Organizations dedicated to PCOS, such as the PCOS Awareness Association, may provide resources and information on support groups. Check their websites or contact them for details on local or online groups.

Meetup Groups:

Meetup.com is a platform where individuals with shared interests, including PCOS, organize local meetups. Search for PCOS-related groups in your area to connect with people in person.

Healthcare Provider Recommendations:

Ask your healthcare provider or specialist if they are aware of any local support groups or resources. They may have insights into groups that align with your specific needs.

Social Media Platforms:

Instagram, Twitter, and other social media platforms often host PCOS advocates and influencers who share experiences and resources. Following relevant accounts can lead you to supportive communities.

Women's Health Organizations:

Women's health organizations may offer support groups or resources for individuals with PCOS. Check with local health organizations or larger entities focused on women's health.

Local Community Centers:

Community centers or health clinics may host support groups for various health conditions, including PCOS. Inquire with local facilities about any existing groups or the potential to start one.

Therapeutic Support Groups:

Some therapists or mental health professionals organize support groups for individuals dealing with conditions like PCOS. These groups often provide a safe space to share experiences and coping strategies.

PCOS Conferences and Events:

Attend PCOS-related conferences, workshops, or events. These gatherings often attract individuals passionate about PCOS awareness and management, providing opportunities to connect.

University Health Services:

University health services or medical centers may organize support groups for various health conditions. Check with nearby universities or teaching hospitals for potential PCOS support groups.

Before joining a support group, consider the format (online or in-person), the group's focus, and whether it aligns with your needs and preferences. Connecting with others who understand the challenges of PCOS can offer valuable insights, emotional support, and a sense of community.

Additional Reading

Certainly! Here are some recommended books and resources for additional reading on Polycystic Ovary Syndrome (PCOS):

"The PCOS Workbook: Your Guide to Complete Physical and Emotional Health" by Angela Grassi:

This workbook provides practical advice on managing both the physical and emotional aspects of PCOS. It includes tools for self-assessment, dietary guidance, and emotional well-being.

"PCOS Diet for the Newly Diagnosed: Your All-In-One Guide to Eliminating PCOS Symptoms with the Insulin Resistance Diet" by Tara Spencer:

Tara Spencer outlines a comprehensive approach to managing PCOS through dietary changes. The book includes meal plans, recipes, and insights into the insulin resistance connection.

"The PCOS Health and Nutrition Guide: Includes 125 Recipes for Managing Polycystic Ovary Syndrome" by Jillian Stansbury and Colleen Dunn:

This guide focuses on nutrition strategies for individuals with PCOS. It includes a variety of recipes and nutritional information to support overall health.

"8 Steps to Reverse Your PCOS: A Proven Program to Reset Your Hormones, Repair Your Metabolism, and Restore Your Fertility" by Fiona McCulloch:

Dr. Fiona McCulloch offers a comprehensive approach to addressing PCOS, covering topics from nutrition and lifestyle to medical interventions. The book provides actionable steps for managing the condition.

"PCOS SOS: A Gynecologist's Lifeline To Naturally Restore Your Rhythms, Hormones, and Happiness" by Dr. Felice Gersh:

Dr. Felice Gersh, a leading expert in PCOS, provides insights into the root causes of PCOS and offers practical advice for managing symptoms naturally.

"Taking Charge of Your Fertility" by Toni Weschler:

While not specific to PCOS, this classic book provides valuable information on understanding and tracking menstrual cycles, which can be beneficial for individuals with PCOS trying to conceive.

"The PCOS Solution: An Evidence-Based Natural Approach to Healing PCOS" by Melissa Diane Smith:

Melissa Diane Smith explores natural approaches to managing PCOS, incorporating dietary recommendations, supplements, and lifestyle changes.

Websites and Establishments:

For further information, articles, and support, visit reliable websites like the American Society for Reproductive Medicine (asrm.org), PCOS Awareness Association (pcosaa.org), and PCOS Challenge (pcoschallenge.org).

Never forget to seek the guidance of medical specialists for personalised recommendations and treatment strategies. These resources can help you better understand PCOS and provide helpful advice on how to effectively manage the illness.

Expert Assistance

In order to effectively manage Polycystic Ovary Syndrome (PCOS), seeking professional assistance is essential. Here are some important experts who can offer advice and support:

Primary Care Physician:

Consult your primary care physician first for a preliminary assessment. They can evaluate your symptoms, perform a physical examination, and, if necessary, recommend you to a specialist.

A gynaecologist:

A gynaecologist is an expert in the reproductive health of women and is capable of diagnosing and treating PCOS. They can offer advice on hormone therapies, issues related to conception, and general gynaecological care.

Endocrinologist:

Hormonal diseases are the specialty of endocrinologists. For a more thorough evaluation, it may be helpful to speak with an endocrinologist if your PCOS symptoms are closely linked to hormone imbalances.

Endocrinologist for Reproduction:

A reproductive endocrinologist is an expert in fertility treatments if that's an issue. They can help with PCOS-related issues related to infertility.

Dietitian or nutritionist:

A qualified dietitian can assist you in developing a customised eating plan that addresses insulin resistance, PCOS symptoms, and promotes general health.

Expert in Mental Health:

Speaking with a mental health expert, such as a psychologist or counsellor, can help with emotional well-being as PCOS can have an affect on mental health.

Exercise specialist or physical therapist:

Working with a physical therapist or exercise specialist can assist in developing a customised exercise programme to address certain health goals, control weight, and enhance insulin sensitivity.

Specialist in Fertility:

A fertility specialist can offer cutting-edge reproductive therapies and advice on assisted reproductive technology if you are having trouble conceiving.

Dermatologist:

A dermatologist can offer specific care and treatment choices for those with skin-related disorders including acne or hirsutism.

Specialist in Sleep:

Sleep problems are occasionally linked to PCOS. It could be helpful to speak with a sleep specialist if you are having problems falling asleep.

A lifestyle coach or health coach:

A health or lifestyle coach can offer advice on how to make long-lasting lifestyle adjustments, such as food adjustments, stress reduction techniques, and regular exercise regimens.

It is crucial to have an honest conversation with a physician about your symptoms, worries, and health objectives. A multidisciplinary team approach can offer complete care for successful

PCOS management. Consistent follow-ups and communication with your medical team are important for your continued wellbeing and support.

CONCLUSION

In summary, managing polycystic ovarian syndrome (PCOS) necessitates a customised and all-encompassing strategy. PCOS management entails a complex journey that includes everything from comprehending the subtleties of the condition to making lifestyle adjustments and getting professional help. Key conclusions are as follows:

Knowledge and Consciousness:

Acquiring knowledge gives one strength. Spend some time learning about PCOS, its signs and symptoms, and how it affects general health. Being aware is the first step in making wise choices and practicing good self-care.

Changes in Lifestyle:

Modifying one's lifestyle is essential for PCOS management. Prioritise stress reduction, a healthy diet, consistent exercise, and enough sleep. Make small, long-lasting changes, and big things can happen.

Expert Advice:

Work together with medical specialists, such as nutritionists, gynaecologists, endocrinologists, and mental health counsellors. Consulting with them guarantees a thorough and customised strategy for managing PCOS.

Assistance Networks:

Make contact with people who have gone through similar things. Communities on the internet, nearby support groups, and advocacy groups provide helpful understanding, camaraderie, and support.

Emotional Health:

Recognise the psychological effects of PCOS. The state of one's mind is crucial to their general health. Prioritise self-care techniques and seek expert advice from mental health specialists when needed.

The state of reproduction and fertility:

Reproductive endocrinologists or other fertility specialists should be consulted if fertility is an issue. In order to ensure a safe pregnancy, talk about family planning, reproductive treatments, and preconception care.

Frequent Observation:

Early detection and management of PCOS symptoms are facilitated by routine check-ups and monitoring. Maintain an active attitude towards your health and be transparent with your medical team.

Tailored Strategies:

Understand that each person's PCOS will present itself in a unique way. One person's solution might not be the same for another. Adapt your strategy to your own demands and situation.

Recall that controlling PCOS is a continuous effort that calls for perseverance and forbearance. People with PCOS can manage their path with confidence and greater well-being by adopting a complete approach, seeking expert help, and cultivating a sense of community.

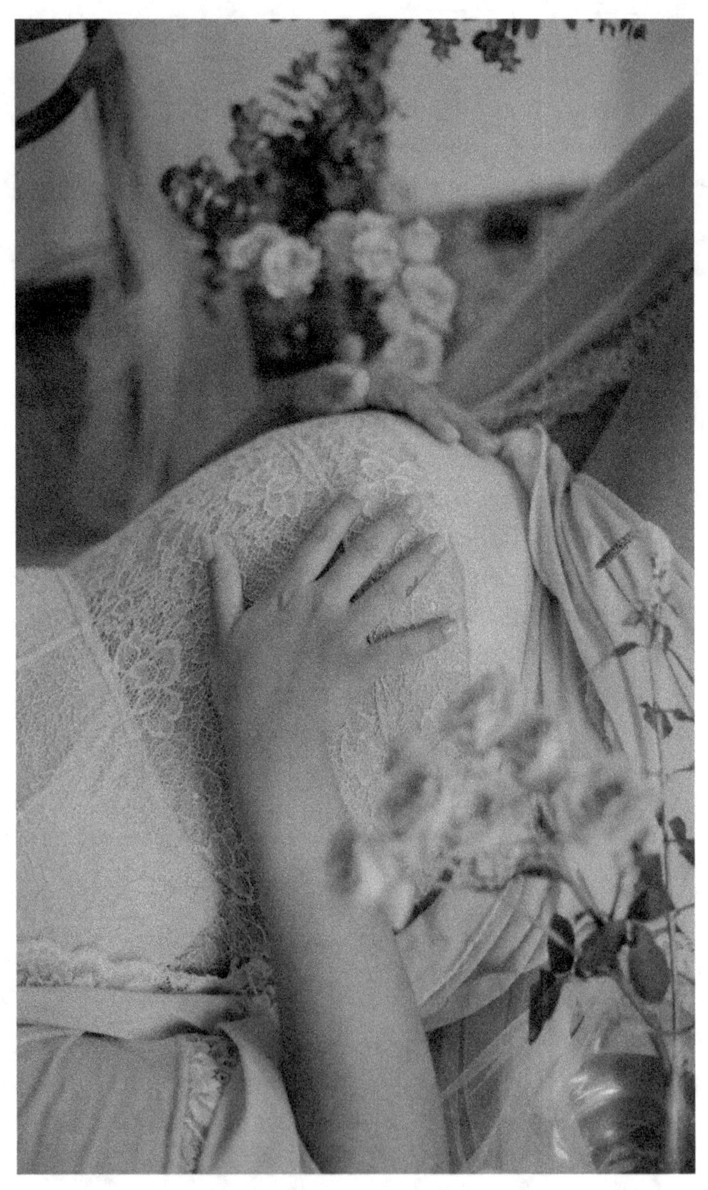